Easy Anemia Diet: Eliminate Iron Deficiency Anemia and low Iron Blood Anemia Naturally

"Discover how you can eliminate Anemia using the food, vitamins and natural remedies."

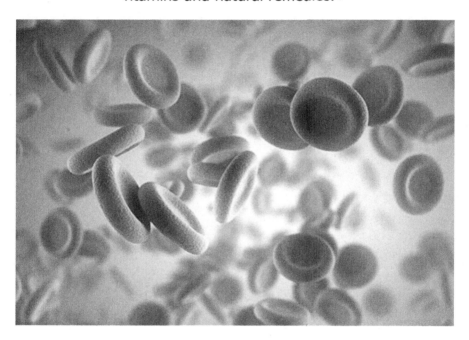

By Rudy S. Silva, Nutritionist

Easy Anemia Diet © 2018 by Rudy S. Silva

Disclaimer and Terms of Use: The Author and Publisher have strived to be as accurate and complete as possible in the creation of this book, notwithstanding the fact that he does not warrant or represent at any time that the contents within are accurate due to the rapidly changing nature of the Internet. While all attempts have been made to verify information provided in this publication, the Author and Publisher assume no responsibility for errors, omissions, or contrary interpretation of the subject matter herein. Any perceived slights of specific persons, peoples, or organizations are unintentional.

Your doctor or health provider should confirm any information given here. This information should not be taken as medical advice or treatment. This e-book is for information and educational purposes only. Consult with your doctor before using any of the foods, remedies or information listed in the book.

Printed in the United States of America, 2018

Table of Contents

1: Anemia Iron Deficiency

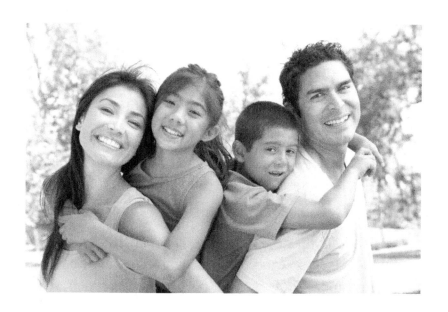

Iron Deficiency Anemia

The most common type of Anemia is Iron Deficiency Anemia, or simply Iron Deficiency. This malady affects over 2.15 billion people worldwide. In the U.S., it is estimated that 30% of the adult population suffers from Iron Deficiency; 66% of which are women of childbearing age as well as children. On the other hand, only 2% of male adults are diagnosed as having Anemia.

Generally, Anemia occurs more frequently in young individuals than with older folks. Nevertheless, people in their 70s and 80s are also likely to suffer from Anemia due to their diminished ability to digest and absorb food.

It is important for older people to rectify this condition as soon as possible. If left unattended, it will result in serious adverse effects on their health that will likely cut short their lives.

Women

Anemia usually occurs in infants, young children, and women.

Teenage girls and pregnant women, in particular, are more prone to anemia. This condition is due to their diet, which, by and large, may be short in iron and in other nutrients that play a role in iron absorption.

Women who go through heavy menstrual periods are also apt to develop Anemia. As women move past their menopausal stage, they seldom become anemic. However, if they do, their Anemia may be a telltale sign of a more serious illness. For instance, these women may be suffering from a bleeding illness, which may appear as Anemia.

Pregnant Women Pregnant and nursing women are also prone to Anemia since their infants require large quantities of iron for their growth and development. Thus, babies who are nursed by iron-deficient mothers are also likely to be anemic.

Iron deficiency is a condition that goes almost unnoticed and undetected so that many anemic individuals are not even aware of their circumstances. More often, they will attribute the symptoms of Anemia to their stressful lives, not knowing that their feeling tired is actually due to Iron deficiency

Children

Children in third-world countries are quite susceptible to anemia. They are typical undernourished and lack the proper nutrients that supply the iron and vitamins necessary for iron absorption. When children are anemic, they are prone to disease, have reduced mental abilities, and are less productive later in life.

It is estimated that iron anemia deficiency is preventing up to 60% of the population, in developing countries, from reaching their maximum mental abilities.

Athletes

Athletes, especially distance and marathon runners, are also found to be susceptible to Anemia. Here, iron is depleted and lost largely through the amount of sweat that they produce, the red blood cells that break down, and the often bleeding the have in the gut. Female athletes are more likely to be afflicted with this condition as compared to males.

Anemia in Elderly

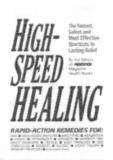

In their book High-Speed Healing, by the editors of prevention, 1991, they talk about anemia in the elderly. "As people age, anemia is more common. Hemoglobin levels often drop in older persons, and they may have problems absorbing iron because they often have less stomach acid, says Paul Stander, M.D. ...Iron-deficiency anemia is not different [in older persons], except that Elderly people don't' tolerate anemia as well," says Dr. Stander, "The elderly can suffer more severe symptoms than younger people for the same amount of anemia."

Anemia Symptoms

Symptoms of iron deficiency include more than just the feeling of being tired and run down. In this book, I will discuss more signs and indications of Anemia. And, I will tell you why irritability and mood swings could be a telltale sign of Anemia.

Nutritional Anemia

Furthermore, studies disclose important details about Anemia.

Among these discoveries, it is revealed that it is not only about the amount of iron that one eats or absorbs that becomes the determining factor in developing Anemia. Rather, it is a matter of the many nutrients that influence the absorption of iron. Hence, shortages of these nutrients will likely result in iron depletion and deficiency.

Add to this, only around 10% of the iron in a good diet is bioavailable.

Health Conditions

Iron plays a vital role in preventing or treating these medical conditions:

- Alcoholism
- Attention Deficit Disorder (ADD)
- Colitis
- Diabetes
- Excessive menstrual blood loss

- Iron Deficiency Anemia
- Leukemia
- Parasitic infections
- Restless leg syndrome
- Stomach ulcers
- Tuberculosis

This makes it more critical that you maintain the proper levels of iron in your blood. Low blood levels point the way to anemia and some of the diseases and conditions mentioned above.

What this book is about

This book will help you assess your condition, whether or not you have Anemia. In most cases, it is important for you to know your condition, so you can immediately address your predicament, or see a doctor if the need arises.

Also, please take note that the intake of iron supplements should be under a physician's direction. Taking iron supplements excessively and without due regard may lead to high levels of iron toxicity, which can result in adverse health effects, or worse, death.

While iron supplements may result in toxicity, natural food sources generally have no side effects, since the iron derived from them is used and absorbed by the body quickly and efficiently. However, there are cases where people have too much iron or iron overload.

For those of you that absorb and accumulate iron in your body, you will have the toxic effects of iron. You will be more susceptible to diabetes, regular headaches, arthritis, extreme tiredness, stomach aches, diarrhea, foggy thinking and many other symptoms. This is a condition called Hemochromatosis, which means you have too much iron in your blood.

In the following chapter, you will learn more about the toxic effects of iron. Though your body uses a variety of ways to absorb and distribute iron, many people are still deficient in iron simply because they do not eat iron-rich food. Most folks eat processed or junk foods that are low in iron.

In addition, they probably don't eat the minerals necessary to help absorb iron. These people fail to eat foods that help circulate blood flow and oxygen throughout their body.

The best way to cure yourself of anemia is to use natural iron found in food and in natural supplements and not chemical substances in pill form, which are imbalanced and result in digestive problems and other unseen side effects.

In this book, I will provide you with information to understand Deficiency Anemia and how to battle it, using natural food and nutrition.

2: How Organic Iron is processed in Your Body

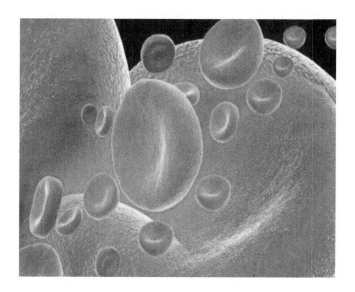

The Role of Iron in Energy Production

Iron has a vital role in the production of energy in your body. As such, iron becomes a constituent of various enzymes iron catalyzes, iron peroxidase and Cytochrome enzymes.

Iron catalase is an enzyme that contains iron. This enzyme is present in every cell and eliminates hydrogen peroxide, as it is created by your cells. Hydrogen peroxide acts as a poison in the cells and reduces the cell's ability to function properly.

As iron levels drop in the blood, iron deficiency occurs in

iron catalase before it drops in the hemoglobin. Iron also helps produce carnitine a non-essential amino acid that aids in the proper use of body fat.

Moreover, your immune system also depends on the availability of iron in the body.

In his book, The Healing Power of Minerals, 1997, Paul Bergner described some of the functions of iron in your body,

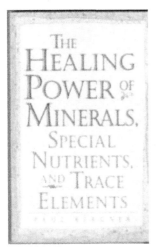

"Most of the body's iron is used to make hemoglobin. Iron is also important in energy release, immune function, and cholesterol metabolism. Myoglobin, which is present in muscles, also contains iron. It helps deliver oxygen and consequently, energy to muscles when they are working hard.

Iron is stored in the liver, spleen, and bone marrow in the form of ferritin, which is used to make more hemoglobin when the need arises. Low levels of ferritin in the blood indicate long-term iron deficiency.

Ironworks in the immune system to fight invading bacteria and viruses. It also assists with detoxification of the liver. Important in the growth process, iron is a constituent in many enzymes and proteins in the body, including the synthesis of DNA."

Iron and Oxygen

Iron is a vital element of the human body. It is essentially found in every human cell and is linked with protein molecules to form hemoglobin. Iron comes in two types - Heme and Non-heme.

Heme Iron can be sourced from animal flesh, while the Non-heme iron is found in fruits, vegetables, and dairy products.

Iron Functions as a Conduit for Oxygen Distribution

Iron is the core of every hemoglobin molecule. Hemoglobin acts as the oxygen-carrying component of each red blood cell.

Accordingly, the ability, of every red blood cell to carry oxygen, depends on the presence of iron.

Deficiency in iron means that the body will likely produce less hemoglobin, which will also result in minimal oxygen distribution throughout your body.

Iron also acts as a constituent of Myoglobin, which is the molecule that holds iron and oxygen. Like hemoglobin, this molecule also acts as an oxygen carrier and distributes oxygen to the muscles and the heart.

Iron Deficiency Anemia is the lack of the mineral iron in your body. It is the depletion of your iron body stores. When you have an iron deficiency, you have a deficiency in hemoglobin.

Your body needs iron to form the hemoglobin molecule since iron is the center of the hemoglobin molecule. Oxygen attaches itself to iron as the hemoglobin molecule passes through your lungs.

The Hemoglobin Molecule

Hemoglobin is a protein molecule that contains an iron center in red blood cells. It is hemoglobin that gives blood its red color. Each red blood cell contains about 20 to 30 million hemoglobin molecules, and each hemoglobin molecule carries with it four iron molecules.

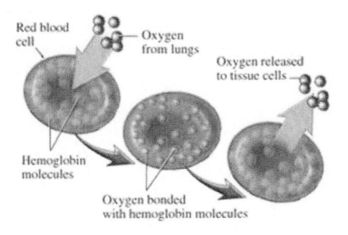

Oxygen is attached to each iron molecule. This means that each red blood cell carries around 800 million to 1.2 billion oxygen molecules.

Hemoglobin Molecule

α chain
iron
heme group
β chain
red blood cell
β chain
α chain
helical shape of the polypeptide molecule

One of the functions of red blood cells is to transport oxygen to all parts of the body and to haul away Carbon Dioxide afterward.

Apparently, every time we inhale, oxygen is picked up by the hemoglobin, and when we exhale the Carbon Dioxide created in your cells is released by your lungs into the air.

If you have Anemia, people may say that you have tired blood.

That's because one of Anemia's symptoms is the feeling of being tired. This condition is largely due to diminished quantities of healthy red blood cells that carry oxygen to the entire body.

Without oxygen, your cells in your body can't burn nutrients that create the needed energy for you to perform your activities. Thus, most anemic individuals feel sluggish and lethargic.

Anemia comes in many forms, with each having its own causes. This illness can also be temporary, or it may run for a long time. Moreover, Anemia can range from mild to serious.

Anemia is a common blood disorder. However, women and people with chronic diseases are at an increased risk of incurring this condition.

Here you can see the part of the cycle of how iron works and travels in your body.

Note the iron is stored in a protein called Ferritin.

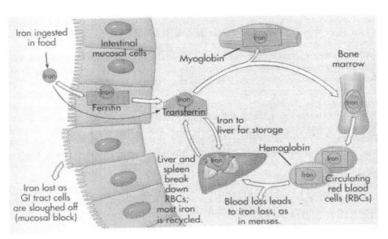

If you suspect you have anemia, see your doctor. Anemia can be a sign of serious illnesses. Treatments for Anemia range from taking supplements to undergoing medical procedures. You may be able to prevent Anemia by eating a healthy, varied diet. Also, taking iron supplements will augment the formation and creation of bioactive iron in the body.

In his book, Food Healing for Man, 1983, Bernard Jensen, Ph. D. writes,

16

"The one element which attracts oxygen from the air, and without which we cannot exist, is iron.

Iron and oxygen are the two frisky horses that work in the body. When you have enough iron, you draw oxygen out of the air; otherwise, you don't get enough oxygen.

When a person gets tired, it is usually an indication of a lack of iron in the body. It is also needed in the metabolism; the activity of the body is dependent upon iron. The best iron sources are black cherries, greens, and chlorophyll. Also, it is high in blackstrap molasses."

3: Diagnosing Anemia

Diagnosing Anemia

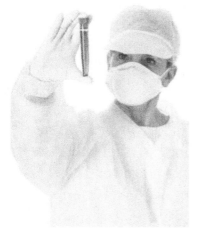

Generally, Anemia is identified and detected through a complete blood count. Using Modern Counters, the number and size of red blood cells, as well as hemoglobin levels, can be determined and recorded.

This type of diagnosis can determine the cause or type of anemia. A microscope inspection of a blood smear is also helpful in diagnosis.

When determining the cause of Anemia proves difficult, as when the cause is not obvious or unapparent, other tests can be performed:

ESR - It is a non-specific test that is used to diagnose conditions associated with cancers, infections, inflammation, and auto-immune diseases, among others.

Although this test does not tell where the inflammation is or what is causing it, ESR can be used in conditions like Anemia, in conjunction with other tests.

Through this test, doctors have a better understanding of what disease they are dealing with.

Ferritin this type of test is deemed the most specific in detecting Iron Deficiency Anemia unless inflammation or infections are also present. Using this method, the blood tests will indicate the levels of hemoglobin, iron and red blood cells, among others.

In his book, Optimum Sports Nutrition, 1993, Dr. Michael Colgan points out,

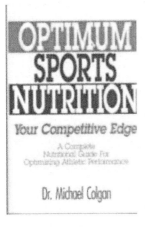

"One of the best marathon runners of all time had a serious iron deficiency. The problem had not shown up in any blood test used by Salazar's medicos, because they were relying on the wrong tests serum iron and hemoglobin. These tests are still wrongly used today by thousands of physicians to diagnose iron deficiency an expert in iron-deficiency, phoned Salazar's coach,

the great Bill Delinger, and suggested he test serum ferritin, an accurate measure of iron stores. The test showed near zero iron."

B Vitamins

Vitamin B12 Deficiency occurs less frequently than Iron

Deficiency, and is generally not caused by dietary deficiency of Vitamin B12. Rather, this disorder is commonly caused by Pernicious Anemia a condition in which the body ceases to produce an intrinsic factor that is essential for the body to absorb Vitamin B12 from the diet.

Vitamin B12 Deficiency causes nerve problems, accompanied by numbness and tingling of the hands and feet. Here, hemoglobin levels are low but the red blood cells are abnormally large.

Folic Acid

Folic Acid Deficiency is similar to Vitamin B12 Deficiency. This disorder can cause certain changes in hemoglobin and red blood cell indices. Usually, folic acid can be found in green, leafy vegetables. In the U. S., folic acid is added in most grain products; hence, its deficiency is rarely the case.

However, there is an increased risk of Folic Acid Deficiency during pregnancy in women. This condition is especially dangerous since folic acid is essential for the growth and development of the baby. Diminished folic acid levels can cause adverse effects on the baby's brain and spinal cord. It is important for pregnant women to take folic acid supplements.

Serum Iron - This medical test measures the amount of iron circulating in the body that is bound to transferrin.

The Serum Iron test is primarily used when doctors are concerned about the likelihood of an iron deficiency in their patients.

The liver produces transferrin. When released, it binds with the iron ions. Transferrin is necessary if the stored iron is used or stored by the body.

Serum Iron Test uses the drawn blood from the veins to measure the iron that is attached to Transferrin and is circulating in the body.

Transferrin - This test comes in many names. Formally, it is known as the Transferrin Saturation Test, or Transferrin, for short.

It is also known as Iron-Binding Capacity Test (IBC), Total Iron-Binding Capacity Test (TIBC) and Serum Iron-Binding Capacity Test, among others.

Transferring Test is frequently used alongside the Serum Iron Test to aid in identifying the likelihood of iron deficiency or overload. This test calculates the transferring saturation:

In iron deficient people, the transferrin saturation is low since iron levels are also low.

In case of iron overload, the iron level is high, but the TIBC is low or normal. In effect, the transferring saturation will increase. Here, an Unsaturated Iron-binding Capacity Test (UIBC) will be conducted instead of TIBC.

When the patient has problems with his liver, it is likely that his transferring levels will also be low.

It is customary to test for transferrin (instead of TIBC or UIBC) when evaluating a patient's nutritional status or liver function. Because it is made in the liver, transferrin will be low in patients with liver disease. Transferrin levels also drop when there is not enough protein in the diet, so this test can be used to monitor nutrition.

When a person suffers from an iron deficiency or overload, a TIBC or UIBC is ordered. More tests may also be ordered if symptoms of Anemia are present.

RBC Folate Level

Folic acid blood testing helps monitor the presence of central nervous system disorders. In addition, this test also helps physicians diagnose Anemia.

Many consider RBC Folate Level Testing more reliable compared to Serum Iron Testing.

Serum Vitamin B12

As its name implies, this test is used to measure the Vitamin B12 level in the blood. Accordingly, it is used to assess vitamin deficiency, which may be caused by poor dietary intake or problems associated with its absorption.

Hemoglobin Electrophoresis

This test is used to check the different types of

hemoglobin present in the blood. Hemoglobin is the substance that transports oxygen throughout the body.

The common types of Normal Hemoglobin are:

Hemoglobin F (Fetal Hemoglobin) This is usually found in newborns, and even in fetuses.

Hemoglobin A (Adult Hemoglobin) It is commonly found in adults. This type replaces Hemoglobin F right after the birth of the child.

Hemoglobin A2 Usually found in small amounts in adults. This is the normal type of hemoglobin.

The Hemoglobin Electrophoresis Test separates the normal hemoglobin from the abnormal types found in the blood. Abnormal hemoglobin may be an indication of a disease. Accordingly, this test helps diagnose the likelihood of Anemia.

Renal Function

This test is used to assess the excretory function of the kidneys since the amount of liquid filtered out by the circulating blood is processed by your kidneys.

4: The Different Anemia's You Might Have

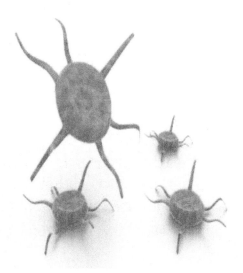

Different Types of Anemia

The size of the red blood cells helps determine the type of the Anemia. If the red blood cells are smaller than 8 fl., the Anemia is considered Microcytic; if it is of normal size, 8 to 10 fl, it is classified as Normocytic; if it is larger than normal, over 10 fl, then it is grouped as Macrocytic.

Microcytic Anemia

Microcytic Anemia is a result of hemoglobin synthesis failure, or the insufficiency thereof. It often results from Iron Deficiency.

In addition, Microcytic Anemia could be caused by:

- Heme Synthesis Defect,

- Iron Deficiency Anemia,
- Globin Synthesis Defect,
- Alpha- and Beta- Thalassemia,
- HbE and HbC Syndrome, and various other unstable hemoglobin diseases,
- Sideroblastic Defect,
- Hereditary or Acquired Sideroblastic Anemia, including Lead Toxicity, and Reversible Sideroblastic Anemia

The most common type of Anemia is Iron Deficiency Anemia. It is also one that has many causes. Here, red blood cells come out paler than usual (hypochromic), as well as appear smaller than regular (microcytic) when viewed under the microscope.

The most common cause of Macrocytic Anemia is Megaloblastic Anemia, which in turn is due to the deficiency of Folic Acid, Vitamin B12 or both. The said deficiency is generally attributable to insufficient absorption or inadequate intake of either or both nutrients.

While Folic Acid Deficiency does not normally produce neurological symptoms, vitamin B12 Deficiency does. Moreover, Vitamin B12 Deficiency causes Pernicious Anemia, which in turn resulted from the lack of intrinsic factor.

Intrinsic factor is required to absorb vitamin B12 from food. A deficiency of intrinsic factor may arise from a condition that targets the parietal cells (atrophic gastritis), which produce intrinsic factor. Accordingly, this will result in the poor absorption of Vitamin B12. The parietal cells are located in the walls of your stomach.

Macrocytic Anemia is also caused by the removal of the functional portion of the stomach during surgery, leading to reduced absorption of Vitamin B12 or folic acid. Thus, one must be aware of his/her affliction of Anemia before undergoing gastric bypass surgery.

William Murphy first discovered the treatment for Anemia caused by Vitamin B12 Deficiency. He first bled dogs to make them anemic, and then fed and nourished these canines to see what would restore their health back to normal. After ingesting large quantities of liver, the dogs seemed to regain their health.

Afterward, George Minot and George Whipple took on Murphy's discovery and proceeded to chemically isolate the Vitamin B12 nutrients from the liver to produce a curative substance.

In 1934, the Nobel Prize in Medicine was shared by Murphy, Minot, and Whipple.

Normocytic Anemia

Normocytic Anemia occurs when the overall hemoglobin levels are decreased, but the red blood cell size remains normal. This condition is generally caused by:

- Acute Hemorrhage blood loss,
- Anemia of chronic disease,
- Aplastic anemia (bone marrow failure),
- Hemolytic anemia.

Dimorphic Anemia

Dimorphic Anemia is a condition that occurs when two causes of Anemia act at the same time. An example would be a Macrocytic Hypochromic, which may be caused by hookworm infestation that leads to a deficiency in iron Vitamin B12 or folic acid. It may also occur when red blood cell indices indicate abnormality following a blood transfusion.

Also, elevated red blood cell distribution width (RDW), which indicates a wider-than-normal red blood cell size, is evidence of multiple causes of Anemia.

Megaloblastic Anemia

When the body is lacking in Vitamin B12, it will give rise to Megaloblastic Anemia. This condition usually occurs in many alcoholics, since alcohol flushes Vitamin B12 out of the body in urine.

Children are generally susceptible to inadequate Vitamin B12, which makes them more prone to Megaloblastic Anemia.

Vegetarians, too, are also at a risk, especially those who do not get much Vitamin B12 in their diet. Accordingly, they need vitamin supplements to avoid developing this type of Anemia.

5: What are The Symptoms of Anemia?

Iron Deficiency Symptoms

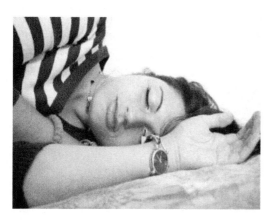

In the U.S., iron deficiency is among the most common nutrient deficiency. This is caused by insufficient dietary intake, parasitic infection, poor absorption of nutrients or other medical conditions. Although the body reuses the iron from old red blood cells to produce hemoglobin for new red blood cells, iron deficiency still causes underdevelopment of red blood cells.

Hemoglobin, Oxygen and Carbon Dioxide

The purpose of the hemoglobin molecule, with iron at its center, is to pick up oxygen in the lungs and transport it to all the cells in your body. And, while at the cells, it will pick up carbon dioxide created by the cells and transport this dioxide back to the lungs for exhalation.

The problem when you don't have enough iron is that there is not enough hemoglobin, so the amount oxygen picked up in the lungs is not enough to supply the body. In addition, when at the cells, hemoglobin cannot pick up all the waste carbon dioxide.

So there occurs a buildup of carbon dioxide in your body. This buildup will cause you to exhibit a variety of symptoms and creates illness and disease when allowing this to continue over a long term.

Pica - Eating Behavior

People with poor iron intake are likely to suffer from Pica, an eating behavior where one eats materials that are inedible, or otherwise unsuitable for consumption, like dirt and soil, among others.

Furthermore, children with iron deficiency also display learning disabilities and low IQ.

The following are symptoms of Anemia:

- Weakness, lethargy, listlessness

- Feeling tired and sluggish
- Loss of stamina
- Increased risk of infections
- Depression
- Apathy
- Low energy
- Shortness of breath
- Increased heart rate
- Headaches
- Sore or smooth tongue
- Sides of mouth crack
- Nausea and loss of appetite

- Dizziness

- Gum bleeding

- Feeling confused, irritability, loss of concentration

- Low tolerance to cold temperature (Iron is needed to create body heat)

- Behavioral disturbances in children

- Rigid, brittle, or spoon-shaped fingernails

- Numbness, tingling, coldness in hands

- Pale skin

- Hair loss

- Stools turn black from the excretion of iron sulfide

- Constipation

- Stomach pain relieved by pressure

- Craving for eating paper, cardboard, dirt, or other substances

- Increase in infections

- Difficulty in swallowing – Dysphagia

Anemia diminishes the capability of anemic individuals to perform physical activities. This is a result of one's muscles being forced to depend on anaerobic metabolism.

Iron Deficiency also causes certain complications, including hypoxemia and brittle fingernails, as well as possible behavioral disturbances in children.

Hypoxemia, caused by Anemia, can worsen the cardiopulmonary condition of patients with the pre-existing chronic pulmonary illness.

On the other hand, low tolerance to cold temperatures may occur only in one out of five patients diagnosed with

Iron Deficiency Anemia. They become manifest through numbness and tingling of the hands.

Other symptoms of Anemia also include fatigue, ranging from mild to extreme. This is likely due to the lack of oxygen in the body.

Eating Paper – Pica

In his book called Trace Elements and Other Essential Nutrients, 2003, Dr. David L. Watts, reports about a patient that craves paper. She ate paper, books and candy wrappings.

This condition is called Pica, which is an abnormal craving for substances other than food. It was this condition that Dr. Watts discovered to be caused by iron deficiency.

Increase in infections

When you lack iron and have nutritional deficiencies, your immune system becomes weaker. If you have a bacterial infection, your body takes the iron in your blood and stores it in your bones, liver, spleen and lymphatic tissues. In this way, the bacteria, which need iron for growth, cannot get the iron it needs.

Since iron becomes stored, it is not available for the hemoglobin. With long-term infections, this can become a real health issue. Infections can be in the body for years, and you don't even know it.

This type of iron deficiency is not curable with the addition of iron to your diet. This disease is called "infectious anemia."

A typical infection can be a dental abscess, which constantly is producing bacteria that move into the blood.

Infectious anemia can be detected, when the iron to copper ratio is high on a TMA test. Once the infection is cleared, iron that is stored will return to the blood, and healing can start to take place.

6: Some of The Causes of Anemia

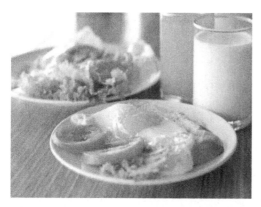

Anemia occurs when there is a deficiency in iron or when the amount of red blood cells or hemoglobin in your body decreases.

It is also brought about when there is a reduction in the amount of blood circulating throughout your body.

Anemia occurs when there is a deficiency in iron or when the amount of red blood cells or hemoglobin in the body decreases. Accordingly, Anemia is brought about by any of these causes:

- Not eating enough foods rich in iron
- Congested and weak liver
- Not having a good healthy diet
- Repeated dieting
- Having a disorder like anorexia nervosa or bulimia
- In babies, breast or bottle feeding is not supplemented
- Rapid growth in children

- Iron malabsorption from having celiac disease and/or chronic diarrhea,
- Blood loss resulting from ulcers, cancer, surgery, injury, gum disease, or bleeding hemorrhoids
- Pregnancy increases the risk of Anemia since iron goes to the fetus
- Pregnancy or heavy menstrual periods
- Prolonged breastfeeding without iron food consumption
- Lack of Vitamin B12, Vitamin C, and folic acid or inability to absorb these vitamins
- Lack of specific minerals, like Copper
- Inherited blood disorders
- Being elderly and having the inability to absorb
- certain, minerals thus affecting iron absorption
- Low levels of stomach acid
- Low levels of an intrinsic factor, which help with B12 adsorption
- Chronic diarrhea
- Gastrectomy – partial or total removal of the lower stomach
- Malaria
- Excess diarrhea
- Respiratory diseases
- Hookworm, trichuriasis
- High Phytates

- Anorexia

Medications That Affect Iron

Certain drugs and medications affect the amount of iron stored in our body:

Aspirin and Non-steroidal Anti-inflammatory medications

medications (e. g. Ibuprofen) may cause gastrointestinal bleeding. This can cause Iron Deficiency Anemia.

Histamine Blockers prevent the release of stomach acid. Drugs like Tagamet, Pepcid, and Zantac, among others, are used to treat ulcers, heartburn and acid reflux and reduce stomach acids. By reducing stomach acidity, these drugs also reduce iron absorption.

Neomycin, an antibiotic, decreases iron levels in your body. Stanozolol is a synthetic anabolic steroid related to testosterone. This drug can cause iron depletion.

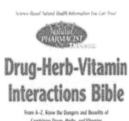

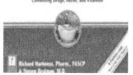

Iron binds with Warfarin (Coumadin), which may decrease Iron Absorption. Penicillamine and Deferoxamine (Desferal) are pharmaceuticals of the chelator class that are used to treat iron intoxication and overload.

In their book called Drug-Herb-Vitamin Interactions Bible, 2000, Richard Harkness, Pharm., FASCP & Steven Bratman, M.D., have these recommendations. If you take

the following drugs, you should not be taking iron pills at the same.

These drugs will have a significant interaction with iron in a **"NEGATIVE [WAY] Take at a Different Time of Day:**

- Ace Inhibitors
- Fluoroquinolones
- Levodopa
- Levodopa/Carbidopa
- Methyldopa
- Penicillamine
- Tetracyclines
- Thyroid Hormone

POSITIVE

Supplementation Possibly Helpful, but Take at a Different

Time of Day:

- Antacids
- Bile Acid Sequestrants
- H2 Antagonists
- Proton Pump Inhibitors"

Furthermore, the use of oral contraceptives results in high levels of iron in the blood, since it significantly reduces the amount of blood lost by women during their menstrual periods.

In their book called The Folk Remedy Encyclopedia, 2001, The editors of FC&A Medical Publishing say that,

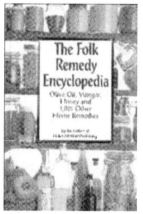

"Pre-menopausal women and people who must take NSAIDs are at greater risk for iron-deficiency anemia. If you have very pale skin, are tired a lot, and have trouble concentrating, you might be low in iron. Some women avoid iron-rich meat to cut calories.

If you don't eat meat, you must replace missing iron with foods like legumes, fortified cereals, and plenty of green leafy vegetables. And be sure to get lots of vitamin C since this vitamin helps you absorb iron better."

Dietary Iron supplements also have the following effects:

Iron binds with Sulfasalazine, decreasing the latter's absorption. Iron supplements also reduce the absorption of tetracycline and thyroid hormone medications. Dietary iron supplements interfere with Carbidopa a drug used for Parkinson's disease treatment. It also decreases the absorption of Methyldopa a drug used to lower blood pressure.

Iron Nutrient Interactions

Vitamin C (Ascorbic Acid), copper, manganese and cobalt increase iron absorption. Amino acids also improve absorption because the acids stimulate the hydrochloric acid in the stomach. However, calcium decreases absorption of dietary iron.

Calcium

The calcium in milk and cheese can slightly inhibit the absorption of iron. This is caused by the high calcium and phosphate content that these dairy products have. It will be a good idea not to take calcium when you know you are eating a high iron meal or when you take an iron supplement.

Cancer and Chemotherapy

Although chemotherapy drugs prescribed by doctors will help destroy cancer cells, they will also destroy the good cells.

For instance, chemotherapy drugs can damage the

bone marrow blood-forming cells thus leading to severe Anemia.

Melatonin and Iron

With the bone marrow cells of St. Petersburg mice, Vladimir Lesnikov conducted tests using various toxic chemotherapy drugs. When these substances were mixed with Melatonin, the damage to the bone marrow was much less than normal.

Based on these findings, chemotherapy sessions conducted at night are found to be more effective and less toxic. Perhaps more Melatonin is in the blood at night.

In the book, The Melatonin Miracle, Walter Pierpaoli, M.D., PH.D., and Williams Regelson M.D., stated that, in fact, many pumps with timers that automatically pulse anticancer drugs into chemotherapy patients were now given intravenously while they slept.

This also means that the treatment did not disrupt normal sleep patterns since melatonin production can be disturbed by the bright lights and noise of a busy hospital.

Saw Palmetto

There are some studies that show that if you are taking the herb Saw Palmetto for benign prostate that it can interfere with the absorption of iron.

Factors That Contribute to Iron Deficiency

The rate of iron absorption increases when the body needs it. This phenomenon is apparent during rapid growth periods in children, and during pregnancy and lactation in women.

People with low stomach acid experience decreased rates of iron absorption. Known as Hypochlorhydria, this condition is common among the elderly, and those who take antacids frequently.

Iron absorption also decreases when one drinks coffee or tea. This is due to this drink's caffeine and tannins content. Thus, people with iron deficiency should wait at least one hour after every meal before drinking green or black tea.

Carbonated soft drinks, which contain phosphates, also reduce iron absorption rates.

Phytates and oxalates may also decrease iron absorption because both elements form complexes with minerals that cannot be absorbed by our digestive system.

Phytates can be found in whole grains, while oxalates are in spinach and chocolate.

Oxalates

Phytates and oxalates may also decrease iron absorption because both elements form complexes with minerals that can not be absorbed by our digestive system. Foods high in oxalic acid are spinach, rhubarb, tomatoes, and chocolate. Phytates can be found in whole grains.

In their book The Hormone Connection, by Gale Maleskey and Mary Kittle with the Editors of Prevention, 2001 say that,

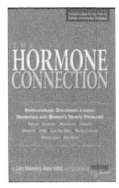

"Heavy bleeding can cause iron deficiency. But the opposite is also true iron deficiency can cause heavier than normal menstrual bleeding, creating a vicious circle that must be stopped, Dr. Shapiro says.

If your periods are heavy and especially if you feel tired and weak,

with shortness of breath and trouble concentrating, see your doctor. Iron Deficiency is easy to detect and treat."

If you're truly anemic, your doctor may initially prescribe large amounts of iron usually in a form called ferrous sulfate. To avoid stomach upset and constipation, some doctors use more readily absorbed form iron succinate or iron fumarate -in small doses several times a day. Some use liver extract, a cholesterol-free liquid that contains other nutrients also needed to rebuild blood such as vitamins B6 and B 12, folic acid, riboflavin, copper, vitamin C, and protein. This approach often resolves anemia better than simply using iron Dr. Shapiro says."

Black Tea

Regular tea or black tea which is high in tannins will inhibit the absorption of nonheme iron, which is found in plants. But by eating those foods – protein and vitamin C - which enhances the absorption of nonheme iron you can neutralize the effects of tannins in regular tea.

To get the benefit of this enhancement, you need to eat or take protein and vitamin C with your meal when you drink your tea.

Copper Deficiency

If your body stores are low in copper or you are not eating enough copper, and you don't need much of it, you will be prone to iron deficiency anemia. Without copper, the hemoglobin in your body will have a hard time bringing in iron into its cells. The excess iron will then be taken up by the various organs in your body.

Despite the excess iron in your body, you will still have anemia. In addition, the excess iron will become toxic in your body causing a variety of other illnesses. The lack of copper works with so many other nutrients that a lack of it can lead to an imbalance of other vitamins and minerals.

7: Anemia Treatments That Are Available to You

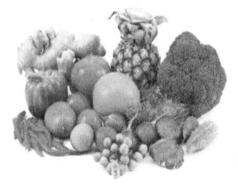

There are many different treatments for Anemia, depending on its severity and causes. Iron deficiency is rare in men and post-menopausal women. In the event of Anemia, the potential causes

would be gastrointestinal bleeding due to an ulcer or colon cancer.

To replenish the diminishing iron in the body, vitamin supplements such as folic acid or Vitamin B12 will do the trick.

In Anemia of chronic diseases, such as those associated with chemotherapy or renal disease, some doctors prescribe recombinant erythropoietin or epoetin alfa to stimulate the production of red blood cells. In case of ongoing blood loss, a blood transfusion may be ordered.

Blood Transfusion for Anemia

As much as possible, doctors will forego blood transfusion as a remedy. Rather, it is deemed as a last resort, since blood transfusion does not necessarily reduce the adverse clinical outcomes. This principle is borne out of the notion that the procedure causes the reduction of oxygen as the number of intensive transfusion strategies increases.

However, in severe bleeding, blood transfusions using donated blood are necessary and life-saving. On the other hand, blood transfusion is deleterious when it comes to an anemic, which appears to be a stable hospitalized patient.

Furthermore, controlled clinical trials reveal that aggressive transfusion strategies resulted in a failure to find beneficial effects. The studies show that instead there are adverse clinical outcomes.

Iron and Hypothyroidism

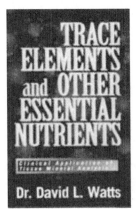

If you have anemia, then you need to know that there is a relationship between anemia and hypothyroidism - abnormally low thyroid hormone production, which causes fatigue, weight gain, depression, sleepiness, dry skin,

decreased concentration, or vague aches and pains.

Dr. David L. Watts of Trace elements and other Essential Nutrients, 1995, says,

"In 1938 physicians discovered a relationship between iron deficiency and hypothyroidism. Cecil stated that both thyroid therapies along with iron therapy were indicated for the treatment of anemia. Today researchers have found that iron deficiency can, in fact, impair thyroid function. The amino acid L-phenylalanine is normally converted to L-tyrosine, which is the precursor to the thyroid hormone thyroxin. It has

46

been found that this conversion is reduced by 50 percent in iron deficient patients. For this reason, low iron stores can be a good indicator for the potential development of low thyroid activity."

Reoccurrence of Iron Deficiency

In the following chapters, various foods, supplements, and herbals are recommended for eliminating lack of iron. It is important to incorporate these diet changes into your normal eating habits.

If you have suffered from an iron deficiency in the past, it can come back. So by following some good eating habits that include iron foods and supplements that enhance iron absorption, you should not have iron deficiency.

No food by itself can give you the amount of iron you need when you are deficient. Getting your iron stores back to normal will takes some time. And the time it takes depends on the severity of your condition.

8: Effects of Iron Poisoning

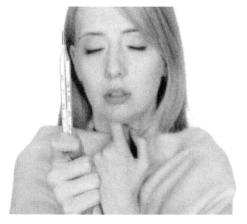

Iron Toxicity

Iron toxicity, or poisoning, is caused when one ingest large quantities of iron. This causes nausea, vomiting, liver failure or damage to the intestinal tract.

Worse, iron toxicity is the leading cause of death in children. Chronic or excessive iron ingestion also causes loss of appetite, headaches, bronze-colored skin and shortness of breath. Here is another list of excess iron in your body:

- Nausea
- Vomiting
- Diarrhea
- Constipation
- Fever
- Severe stomach pain

The effects of excess iron relate to the whole body. In the brain iron through various chemical reactions causes the creation of free radicals, which damage brain cells.

Just like other heavy metals – lead, mercury, and cadmium - Excess iron acts like a free radical causing tissue damage as it travels travel throughout your body.

In the right amounts, iron is required for brain growth and development. It regulates many brain hormones, like neurotransmitters, serotonin, and dopamine.

It is critical that in your efforts to increase the consumption of iron and your stores of iron that you monitor your progress with your doctor. If you are taking iron pills and practicing many of the food principles listed in this book, the doctor will surely monitor your progress. In this way, you will not approach the level of "iron overload" in your body.

Blood Transfusions

Iron toxicity usually occurs only in people who regularly go through blood transfusions, take excessive iron supplements or those diagnosed with Hemochromatosis.

Iron overload is not likely to result from natural food sources.

In hemochromatosis, iron is deposited in the tissues, particularly in the liver, pancreas and the heart; thus, resulting in diabetes, cirrhosis or cardiac insufficiency.

Men are a greater risk of iron toxicity since they do not experience that much iron loss compared to women. Accordingly, men are prone to heart diseases and cancer due to excessive iron.

In addition, iron toxicity is also associated with rheumatoid arthritis.

In some research studies, excess iron has been linked to cancer.

Iron overload

Getting too much iron in your body is extremely detrimental to your health. Excess body iron is more common in men and children. Children can get an overload of iron when they find iron pills and swallow them. Put these pills up high where children can't get them.

So where do men or women get overloaded with iron? Here is a list of sources of iron. When taken in excess can put more iron in your body than needed.

Cooking all your food in iron pots

Drinking water where the soil is high in iron

Drinking water from old homes with old iron pipes

Drinking filtered water where a carbon filter not replaced regularly

Using and drinking herbal teas high in iron in excess – peppermint, chickweed, comfrey root, licorice root, goldenseal In Trace Elements and Other Essential Nutrients, Dr. David L. Watts, tells us that,

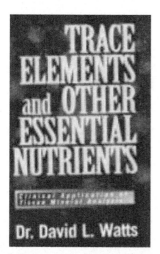

"Alcohol is known to increase iron absorption. Excess iron is known to contribute to cirrhosis of the liver, which is common with alcoholism. Certain beverages are high in iron as well, for example, red wines and imported dark beers.

51

This may be why many people get headaches when they drink dark wines, but do not suffer if they drink white wine, which is low in iron."

In his book called Iridiagnosis, 1985, Henry Lindlahr M. D. talks about how your iris can show if you have an excess of iron in your body. He talks about the iris image shown below,

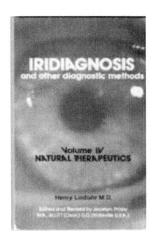

"We find that iron after it has been taken in considerable quantities in the inorganic form shows in the areas of the stomach and bowels as rust brown discoloration which closely resembles the color of iron rust. I have verified this sign in hundreds of cases in people who had absorbed iron in an inorganic form in medicines or in water strongly impregnated with the mineral." He continues and discusses one of his cases.

"The area around [her] pupil corresponding to the region of the stomach and intestines showed a very heavy [brown] iron discoloration for several years she had used water from the iron spring in Lincoln Part. After forming this habit she had suffered much from constipation and indigestion."

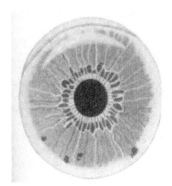

The brown area appears as little droplets circling on top of white rings that borders the black pupil. (see diagram 1) An excess of iron has also been linked to chronic

constipation. It is also known to be linked to colorectal cancer.

Diagram 1: an excess storage of iron in your body. While iron supplements may result in toxicity, natural food sources generally have no side effects, since the iron derived from them is used and absorbed by the body quickly and efficiently.

Stools

When you have an excess of iron in your body, your stools may turn a dark green or black. In addition, you may suffer from constipation. If you are normal, you will have one to two bowel movements every day. If you are constipated, you will have a bowel movement every two to three days. Some people may have a bowel movement every four to five days – consider this severe constipation.

Normal stools are light brown and continuous. If yours are in short pieces, then you lack fiber in your diet. Your stools should float and not sink to the bottom of the toilet bowl.

When you go to the bathroom for a bowel movement, you should only be there for about three to five minutes. If you have to push and strain to get your stools out, then you are constipated.

9: What to Eat When You Have Anemia

Iron from Meat

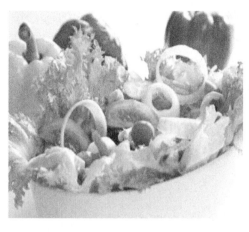

Heme iron, from meat, is up to 15 times more absorbable than other types of iron. When you eat meat, you can absorb up to 25 to 30% of the heme iron content.

Also, the protein in meat enhances this absorption. When eating nonheme iron 2 to 20 % of this iron is absorbed.

It has been found that by adding some meat to stir-fried vegetables or raw salads, the absorption of nonheme iron in the vegetables is enhanced.

One thing to know is when you eat chicken, or poultry, the dark meat has an increase in iron, because the red hemoglobin makes the meat darker.

Canned clams and oysters are also high in iron. Four oz of turkey, dark meat, has as much iron as 1 cup of prune juice.

Fruits and Vegetables

A diet consisting of fruits, vegetable, legumes, nuts, and grains provide enough iron for the body. Vitamin C-rich foods and drinks enhance iron absorption.

Other good sources of iron include broccoli, Swiss chard, and other green leafy veggies. Iron-fortified cereals, pasta, rice, enriched bread, soybean, and blackstrap molasses are also good sources of iron.

Dairy products, like milk, are extremely low in iron. In addition, they interfere with iron nutrition, especially in small children. So avoid these food products until you overcome your anemia. Dr. Neal Pinckney, at The Healing Heart Foundation, says that vegetarian diets high in Vitamin C and Ascorbic acid increases iron absorption from two to six times more.

Foods That Contain Iron

Most foods have little iron content. However, meat has a good amount of iron (heme iron). Other foods high in iron include dulse, kelp, and rice bran. You may also want to check out blackberries, raisins, black walnuts, prunes, figs, black cherries, spinach and other dried fruits.

Food Sources of Iron

Excellent Sources-Very Good Sources-Good Sources

Chard	Romaine Lettuce
Beef Tenderloin	Spinach
Blackstrap Molasses	Lentils
Thyme	Shiitake Mushrooms
Brussels sprouts	Turmeric
Tofu	Asparagus
Dried Beans	Mustard Greens

Venison   Turnip Green

Garbanzo beans   String beans

Broccoli   Leeks

Kelp

Iron is extremely volatile. Cooking these vegetables will eliminate its iron content by as much as 50%.

More people suffer from iron deficiency due to the low iron content of the food they eat. Most food products nowadays are processed, which degrades its nutritional value. Some foods that are overly cooked result in the elimination of whatever iron are in them.

People with arthritis, cold hands and feet, or having low energy are likely to be iron deficient. Using these natural remedies and iron supplements will help increase your body's iron levels, and in due time, you will recover from Anemia.

In 2000, the Institute of Medicine at the National Academy of Sciences established an Adequate Intake level for infants up to six months old and the recommended dietary allowances for all other age categories.

The recommendations appear as follows:

Age Recommended Dietary Allowance

0-6 months	0.27mg
7-12 months	11mg
1-3 years	7mg
4-8 years	10mg

Boys, 9-13 years	8mg
Boys, 14-18	11mg
Girls, 9-13	8mg
Girls, 14-18	15mg
Men, 19-30	8mg
Men, 31-50	8mg
Men, 51-70	8mg
Men over 70	8mg
Women, 19-30	18mg
Women, 31-50	18mg
Women, 51-70	8mg
Women over 70	8mg
Pregnant, 14-50	27mg
Lactating, 14-18	10mg
Lactating, 19-50	9mg

Since iron status is influenced by the type of diet consumed, and by oral contraceptives, the Institute of Medicine established more recommendations for vegetarians, and also for women taking oral contraceptives.

Allowance

Adult male (vegetarian), 14 mg

Adult, premenopausal female (vegetarian),33 mg

Adolescent girl (vegetarian), 26 mg

Adolescent girls taking oral contraceptives, 11.4 mg

Adult, premenopausal women & oral contraceptives, 10.9 mg

Iron

Women and teenage girls need iron at least 15 mg. each day. Men, on the other hand, only need around 10 mg.

Children need to have 10 to 12 mg. of iron every day, preferably sourced from their diet. Generally, breastfeeding is the best source of iron for babies.

But the most at risk of being iron deficient are pregnant women, adolescent girls, and infants.

Infants who are iron deficient are also likely to have impaired learning abilities, as well as having behavioral problems. Iron deficiency can also affect the infant's immune system, and cause fatigue and weakness.

Vitamin C aids in the absorption of iron. Thus, it is wise to eat foods rich in it while also taking in iron supplements.

Tannin in herbal tea, however, hinders the absorption of iron.

Iron supplements tend to neutralize the effects of Vitamin E. It is best to take both at different times of the day so as not to waste the beneficial effects of the other.

A note to all vegetarians: You need to get twice as much iron in your diet compared to meat eaters.

Fruits and Vegetables Rich in Iron

Getting the kids to eat vegetables can be a challenging task. Instead of having to force-feed them every meal time, why not let them take snacks frequently during the day.

Raisins are considered the best source of iron for kids.

They can munch on raisins, whether they are playing with the toys or reading their books. It's a fun approach to iron supplementation for kids.

The best sources of iron are lean meat, beans, tofu and cream of wheat cereal, a cup of Kellogg's Most, and a cup of Kellogg's Product 19, a cup of Total, and a cup of Kix.

There are many other cereals that have good iron content:

Bran Buds, Buck Wheat, Cheerios, Grape Nuts Flakes,

Honey Bran, Special K, Wheat Chex, and Wheaties.

The one thing about too much fiber, which can be obtained by eating these high fiber cereals, is that they inhibit nonheme iron absorption.

The fiber in seeds and grains like wheat, oats, and flaxseeds have a chemical called phytic acid. Phytic acid binds with minerals such as zinc, iron, and calcium, which then go out in your stools.

So phytic acid bind with nonheme iron. But its ok to eat various fiber cereals, but don't go overboard. So don't consume more than 20 to 25 grams of fiber with a low iron diet.

One fiber that does not bind with minerals is the fiber found in coconut meat. The use of all the coconut products such as coconut water, meat, oil, and milk can bring you more balance to your body's chemistry. It can build up your immune system and can help to decrease any loss of blood that you might have throughout the body.

One thing to know about iron-fortified cereals is that the iron they contain is not always very absorbable.

Always use some form of fruit when eating cereal to provide vitamin C and trace minerals, making the iron more absorbable. Drinking a good vitamin C drink will also be helpful. You can also eat a high vitamin C fruit after your cereal.

Look at the fruit list below. And do not eat a lot of cereals that contain bran as this fiber food interferes with iron absorption.

Fruits that are rich in Iron include:

Black and red raspberries and their juices, Grapes, Strawberry, black or red cherries Tomatoes, Kiwi, Bananas

Vegetables that are rich in iron include:

Lima Beans, Peas, Mushrooms

Potatoes, Sweet Potato, Carrots, Corn

Squash – winter, Squash – summer, Avocado

Spinach, Broccoli, Kale

Kidney beans

Dried Fruits with Iron

Here are the best-dried fruits and seeds to eat for iron:

Dried apricots, dried peaches, pumpkin seeds, sunflower seeds

Other excellent sources of iron include chard,

turmeric, spinach, and thyme.

Vegetable Juices with Iron

Here is a drink you can make if you have a juicer. Place into a juicer 3 beet tops, 5 carrots with no green tops, green pepper, and one apple. The apple juice will make this drink more palatable.

Foods high in iron help improve oxygen and blood circulation throughout your body. It also keeps your immune system in tip-top condition. High-Iron foods also provide your body with its much-needed energy.

Vegetables and Fruits high in iron

Dark green	Alfalfa
Spinach	Watercress
Green onions	Kale
Broccoli	Chard
Squash	Okra
Carrots	Radishes
Beets	Yams
Tomatoes	Potatoes

Bananas	Apples
Dark grapes	Apricots
Raisins	Plums
Strawberries	Sunflower seeds
Black beans	Sesame seed
Leafy lettuce	Peas
Egg yokes	Honey
Black cherries	Red cherries
Black strap Molasses	

In many instances, people come to me and ask, "I have anemia, what do I eat so I can get more iron?"

What I tell them is that foods having a large supply of organic iron are hard to find. However, organic iron is the type of iron you should take since it is not toxic for your body. Typically, the food you should eat is one that provides you with iron, oxygen, and magnesium.

First off, your diet should consist of alkaline foods. You should be eating 80% alkaline ash food and 20% acid ash food. Ash foods are those that turn into alkaline or acid residues after they are digested by your cells. Accordingly, you should concentrate on eating raw fruits and vegetables, which are high in iron.

Bananas have folic acid and Vitamin B12. Honey is rich in copper, which is necessary for iron assimilation. Sunflower seeds contain almost as much iron as the liver.

Typically, the liver is prescribed for Iron Deficiency Anemia. However, its toxicity depends on how the animal was fed, bred or preserved.   Only use liver that comes from animals that were raised and fed on non-toxic food, and processed without nitrite and other preservatives.

Remember:

Whenever possible, go organic. Eat fruits and vegetables.

Apricots which are rich in cobalt are excellent for building the blood.

Black Strap Molasses

Another food that has been found high in natural iron is Black Strap Molasses. As mentioned in Dr. Bernard Jensen's book, Food Healing for Man, it is high in iron and calcium. Molasses is high in minerals and various nutrients.

Using two teaspoons or tablespoons per day can help you bring your hemoglobin count back to normal and in

the range of 14 to 18 gm/dl.

In his book, Crude Black Molasses, 1968, Cyril Scott writes,

"   Considering the amount of assailable iron and calcium in Molasses, it is not surprising to hear that many cases of anemia have been cured by taking the [molasses.]   The orthodox treatment of anemia, which consists largely in the administration of some preparation of iron in large does for a long time is not only unsatisfactory but is often attended with unpleasant results in the form of digestive disturbances. The reason is obvious to all naturopaths, for iron and calcium should be absorbed from some natural food and not from some medicinal preparation."

One thing to keep in mind is that all fruits and vegetable that are red or are deep or dark red help to build your blood.

Vegetable Juices

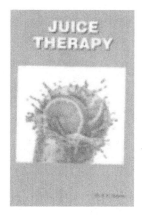

Juices made from fresh vegetables like spinach, alfalfa, watercress, parsley or wheat grass are good for your body. You can also mix these up with carrot and red beet juice or some apple juice. Doctors recommend drinking two glasses a day. Dr. S.K. Sharma, in his book, Juice Therapy, 2007, recommends spinach juice for anemia.

Here what he says, "Since it is a storehouse of iron, it is very useful for removing anemia (even the pernicious variety), constipation, nervous disorders. Give juice of spinach daily to a pregnant woman who often is found to have low iron-deficiency, it will make up for the lost blood, impoverished blood will be richer, and generally, the health of the mother and the baby will also be improved.

It is a natural way to compensate for lassitude of ferrous sulfate. Since its iron release is sustained, it is absorbed gradually and easily digested. In certain sensitive persons, spinach juice disturbs the digestive system, sometimes causing diarrhea or black stools [if so, then] dilute the pure juice with water."

Other juices to drink are prune, apricot, red grape, black currant, and blueberry.

An Iron Tonic

Here is what is called an iron tonic. Take 8 oz of tomato juice, squeeze the juice of one lemon into it, then add three tablespoons of unflavored gelatin powder and two tablespoons of desiccated liver. Mix this up and drink first thing in the morning about 1 hour before breakfast. And also drink one glass before lunch and dinner.

This is a powerful iron drink that provides heme iron from the liver, protein from gelatin and vitamin C from the lemon and tomato to enhance adsorption of the heme iron.

Food and Drinks to Avoid

The International Center for Control of Nutritional Anemia, in cooperation with the University Of Kansa Medical Center, discovered that the following foods and drinks interfere with the absorption of iron in your body:

Do not drink tea or coffee with your meat meals, or within two hours after your meal. They can reduce the absorption of iron from 40 to 66%. Coffee consumption at least one hour before a meal does not inhibit iron absorption.

Do not eat soy or soy flour products. It contains both enhancing and inhibiting iron factors. As much as possible, avoid these.

Avoid eating legumes such as soybeans, black beans, lentils, split peas, and mung beans. They only allow 1-2% of the iron they contain to be absorbed. Most vegetables allow about 10% of their iron to be absorbed.

Dairy products and eggs also reduce the absorption of non-heme iron. However, they do not interfere with the absorption of heme iron.

Oxalates found in certain foods have also been found to limit the amount of iron absorbed into your body. But they only interfere with the iron found in them, and not of that in other foods eaten at the same time. A diet high in wheat bran can interfere with the absorption of iron. Have a diet that is mixed with other grain fibers.

If you are low in iron, try to avoid this food and drinks as much as possible.

How Does Cooking, Storage, and Processing Affect Iron?

Iron can be found in whole grains. Nevertheless, the milling processing takes about 75% of the iron found in it. Refined grains, on the other hand, are usually fortified with iron. However, the added iron is less absorbable compared to the natural iron fund in whole grains.

In addition, take heed of the cookware used. Cast iron pots and pans can add iron to the food cooked in them. If you don't eat a lot of meat or are a vegetarian, then getting iron this way could be helpful.

However, be aware that this practice will eventually lead to iron toxicity, so only use this technique to add more iron to your diet, when you need it. But, also know that this type of iron is not that well absorbed by your body.

Vegetarians

If you are a vegetarian, do not depend on the legumes for your iron.

Many vegetarians usually have normal amounts of hemoglobin. But it has been found that they lack good iron stores in their body. They lack the iron ferritin in the muscles, liver, and bone marrow.

Nutrient Rating System Chart

The Nutrient Rating System Chart will help identify foods and their corresponding nutrients or calories. This system allows highlighting the nutrient content of various foods.

Using the following chart, you can calculate the food's nutrient content. For the nutrient ratings, the standard used are those adopted by the U. S. Food and Drug Administration in their "Reference Values for Nutrition Labeling.

Foods that are ranked high in Iron

Food	Serving, Amount	High in Size (Mg)	Foods Iron Rating
Thyme, dried, ground	2 Tsp	3.56	excellent
Dill weed	2 Tsp	0.98	very good
Cumin seeds	1 Tsp	1.32	very good
Parsley, fresh	2 tsp	0.46	good

Basil, dried, ground	2 Tsp	1.28	very good
Spinach, boiled	1 cup	6.43	excellent
Oregano, dried, ground	2 Tsp	1.32	very good
Cinnamon, Ground	2 tsp	1.72	very good
Turmeric, Powder	2 tsp	1.88	excellent
Black Pepper	2 tsp	1.24	very good
Swiss chard, boiled	1 cup	3.96	excellent
Rosemary, dried	2 tsp	0.64	good
Romaine lettuce	2 cup	1.23	very good
Blackstrap Molasses	2 tsp	2.39	very good
Tofu, raw	4 oz-wt	6.08	very good
Kelp (sea vegetable)	0. 25 cup	0.57	good
Coriander seeds	2 tsp	0.56	good
Mustard greens, boiled	1 cup	0.98	very good
Shiitake mushrooms, raw	8 oz-wt	3.59	very good
Turnip greens, cooked	1 cup	1.15	very good
Green beans, boiled	1 cup	1.6	very good

Leeks, boiled	0.50 cup	0.57	good
Kale, boiled	1 cup	1.17	good
Broccoli, Steamed	1 cup	1.37	good
Shrimp, steamed/boiled	4 oz-wt	3.5	good
Brussels sprouts, boiled	1 cup	1.87	good
Asparagus, boiled	1 cup	1.31	good
Soybeans, Cooked	1 cup	8.84	good
Olives	1 cup	4.44	good
Lentils, Cooked	1 cup	6.59	good
Venison	4 oz-wt	5.07	good
Pumpkin seeds, raw	0.25 cup	5.16	good
Sesame seeds	0.25 cup	5.24	good
Celery, raw	1 cup	0.48	good
Quinoa, Uncooked	0.25 cup	3.93	good
Fennel, raw, sliced	1 cup	0.64	good
Chili pepper, dried	2 tsp	0.6	good
Kidney beans, cooked	1 cup	5.2	good
Mustard seeds	2 tsp	0.76	good

Tomato, ripe	1 cup	0.81	good
Lima beans, cooked	1 cup	4.49	good
Pinto beans, cooked	1 cup	4.46	good
Green peas, boiled	1 cup	2.46	good
Crimini mushrooms,raw	5 oz-wt	0.57	good
Summer squash, cooked, sliced	1 cup	0.65	good
Beets, Boiled	1 cup	1.34	good
Garbanzo beans cooked	1 cup	4.74	good
Collard greens, boiled	1 cup	0.87	good
Navy beans, cooked	1 cup	4.51	good
Beef tenderloin, lean, broiled	4 oz-wt	4.05	good
Black beans, cooked	1 cup	3.61	good
Calf's liver, braised	4 oz-wt	2.97	good
Sweet potato, baked, w/skin	1 each	1.46	good

Iron content of Foods, Milligrams per 100 grams edible portion

Type of Food	Iron Content Mg
Dulse	150
Kelp	100
Rice bran	19.4
Rice polish	16.1
Wheat bran	14.9
Pumpkin & Squash	11.2
Sesame seed, whole	10.5
Wheat germ	9.4
Irish moss	8.9
Soybean, dried	8.4
Pigeon pea, dried	8.0
White bean, dried	7.8
Lima bean, dried	7.8
Hot red pepper, dry	7.8
Mung bean, dried	7.7

Pistachio nut	7.3
Sunflower seed	7.1
Broad bean, dried	7.1
Red bean, dried	6.9
Chickpea, dried	6.9
Butternut	6.8
Lentil, dried	6.8
Millet	6.8
Pinto bean, dried	6.4
Agar	6.3
Parsley	6.2
Peach, dried	6.0
Black walnut	6.0
Cowpea, dried	5.8
Apricot, dried	5.5
Longan, dried	5.4
Pinon nut	5.2

Pea, dried	5.1
Almond	4.7
Prune, dehydrated	4.4
Sorghum, grain	4.4
Durum wheat	4.3
Wild rice	4.2
Prune, dried	3.9
Cashew nut	3.8
Rye grain	3.7
Raisin	3.5
Purslane leaves	3.5
Wheat, soft winter	3.5
Brazil nut	3.4
Filbert	3.4
Pilinut	3.4
Jerusalem artichoke	3.4
Wheat, hard winter	3.4

Chestnut, dried	3.3
Coconut meat, dry	3.3
Beet greens	3.3
Swiss chard	3.2
English walnut	3.1
Dandelion greens	3.1
Spinach	3.1
Wheat, hard spring	3.1
Mustard greens	3.0
Date	3.0
White wheat	3.0
Fig, dried	3.0
Banana Dehydrated	2.8
Tamarind	2.8
Lima bean, fresh	2.8
Soybean, fresh	2.8
Fennel	2.7

Kale leaves	2.7
Barley, scotch pearled	2.7
New Zealand spinach	2.6
Persimmon, native	2.5
Swamp cabbage	2.5
Sesame seed, hulled	2.4
Hickory nut	2.4
Pecan	2.4
Cowpea, fresh	2.3
Kale leaves & stems	2.2
Peanut	2.1
Macadamia nut	2.0
Lettuce: Boston, Bibb	2.0
Pea, fresh green	1.9
Jujube, dried	1.8
Coconut cream	1.8
Turnip greens	1.8

Lychee, dried	1.7
Olive, ripe mission	1.7
Coconut meat, fresh	1.7
Chestnut, fresh	1.7
Chive	1.7
Endive (escarole)	1.7
Watercress	1.7
Apple, dried	1.6
Elderberry	1.6
Granadilla	1.6
Olive, green pickled	1.6
Olive, ripe ascolano	1.6
Olive, ripe sevillano	1.6
Coconut milk	1.6
Dock (sorrel)	1.6
Pigeon pea, fresh	1.6
Brown rice	1.6

Carambola	1.5
Brussels sprouts	1.5
Collard leaves	1.5
Garlic	1.5
Mustard spinach	1.5
Salsify	1.5
Horseradish, raw	1.4
Lettuce: dark looseleaf	1.4
Artichoke, globe	1.3
Cress	1.3
Mung bean sprouts	1.3
Pea, dried	1.3
Breadfruit	1.2
Loganberry	1.2
Longan, fresh	1.2
Roseapple	1.2

Canned oysters are one of the highest foods in iron. For a snack combine this food with whole grain crackers. Eating the red or Manhattan variety clam chowder gives you plenty of iron.

10: Natural Herbal Remedies That Give Your Iron

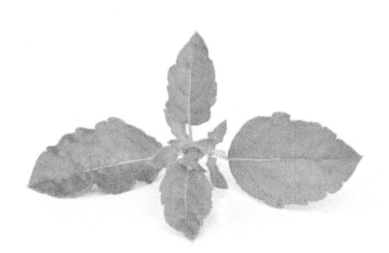 In an att em pt to eli mi nat e an em ia, it is always best to use food or natural remedies. The use of iron supplements or drugs to increase the blood iron levels have their limitations and may prove ineffective for long-term programs.

Using iron supplements always has to be done under a doctor's care because of the toxicity of excessive iron in your body. Iron, given as a supplement, such as ferrous sulfate, is not a balanced chemical, whereas food that contains iron is balanced, with other minerals and nutrients by nature.

The result of this balance is that you will absorb more iron and there is no issue with iron toxicity. So, no matter how much food you eat that is high in iron, that is provided your body organs are working properly.

The other problem with ferrous sulfate is that it has side effects such as constipation; darkened or green stools; diarrhea; nausea; stomach upset.

Seek medical attention right away if any of these SEVERE side effects occur, when using Ferrous Sulfate:

Severe allergic reactions (rash; hives; itching; difficulty breathing; tightness in the chest; swelling of the mouth, face, lips, or tongue); black, tarry stools; blood or streaks of blood in the stool; fever; vomiting with continuing sharp stomach pain.

This is not a complete list of all side effects that may occur. If you have questions about side effects, contact your health care provider.

Types of Iron

There are two types of iron Heme and Non-heme. Heme Iron is found in meat and is generally bio-available. Moreover, heme iron is an absorbable form of iron at 33% more than non-heme iron.

Sources of non-heme iron include fruits and vegetables. To utilize this type of iron, the body needs to ionize and chemically change it. If the body lacks the ability to do so, it will not be able to gain the maximum benefit from this.

On a side note, non-heme iron is prone to blockage from fiber, phosphates, tannates, calcium, and preservatives.

Herbs to Use

To fight off disease, we need to fortify our bodies. One of the ways to do so is to cleanse our bodies from its waste. Much of it comes in the form of mucoid plaque. While taking in pharmaceuticals may seem convenient, given our busy everyday lives, herbs are far more beneficial in the long run.

Herbs can effectively clear out the toxins in the body. Herbs loosen the mucoid plaque, which in turn strengthens our bodies against disease.

Along with the proper diet and exercise, these herbs will cleanse your bodies:

Black Currant

With its strong scent, the blackcurrant is widely used for various medicinal purposes. This herb grows in Scotland's damp woods and is considered as a native of Yorkshire and the Lake District.

Its leaves have cleansing and diuretic properties while its roots are useful against eruptive fevers. When used as a tea, black currant is a perfect medication for inflammatory sore throats.

Burdock Root

Burdock, like Dandelion, is considered a blood purifier, which has plenty of different nutrients that can build the body. It cleanses the blood by removing impurities and harmful acids very quickly. It is a good source of iron and can be used for treating iron.

Chaparral

Chaparral has blood purifying chemicals, which also help to renew the blood and give it a chance to build its strength back up.

In the book called 10 Essential Herbs, 1992, Lalitha Thomas tells how Chaparral helps to eliminate anemia,

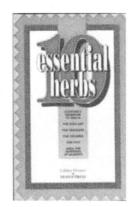

"Chaparral also contains a small amount of the trace element molybdenum. This trace element is known for enhancing hemoglobin formation and is wise to use in conjunction with easy to assimilate iron supplements and with herbs high in iron, such as Comfrey.

For blood building as opposed to blood purifying, Chaparral is most often mixed with other blood building herbs, such as Slippery Elm and Comfrey. "

Dandelion

For centuries, dandelion has been used for detox purposes. It is particularly used for cleansing the liver. It is a rich source of Vitamin A, potassium, calcium, phosphorus, potassium and iron.

Fenugreek

As a diaphoretic, fenugreek has cleansing effects as it helps the body sweat out the toxins. Accordingly, the scent of fenugreek can be smelled on the skin and underarms; much like garlic, though it is not as offensive as the latter.

Fenugreek is also known as a lymphatic cleansing herb. It acts as a vacuum cleaner for the body since its vital role is trapping toxins, trapped proteins, and dead cells. It also stimulates and strengthens the immune system of the body.

Raspberry Leaves

Various researchers reveal that raspberry leaves are helpful for pregnant women since it strengthens the female reproductive system, particularly the wall of the uterus. This herb alleviates nausea and morning sickness.

It is also known for helping prevent hemorrhaging during labor. It also increases milk for lactation.

Raspberry leaves also decrease the profuse menstrual flow. It soothes the bowels, as well as stomach aches. High in vitamins and minerals, raspberry tea is mild and has a pleasant taste.

Kelp

Rich in iodine, kelp promotes thyroid functions. It works wonderfully for the growth, energy, and metabolism in the body.

Kelp is also rich in iron, potassium, and calcium, all of which helps women during menstruation, while pregnant or when nursing their child.

This herb regulates the pituitary glands and is particularly beneficial for nail and hair growth. In addition, kelp also helps normalize the body temperature.

Moreover, kelp is good for the pancreas and the prostate. It promotes the growth of the cell membranes. It cleanses the body from radiation, prevents tumors, and regulates glands and hormones.

Angelica or Dong-Quai

Traditional Chinese medicine uses Angelica to cleanse the arteries and promote blood circulation throughout the body.

Also known as dong-quai, this herb is used to treat Anemia and weak glands, regular monthly periods, and correct hot flashes and vaginal spasms.

For severe conditions, take two capsules of dong-quai two to three times per day. For less severe conditions, useless. You can pop open these capsules and add their contents to your soups or salads since its taste is not bitter.

Side effects of Dong-quai or Angelica

Do not use dong-quai if you have bleeding disorders, excessive menstrual bleeding, diarrhea or a cold or flu. Dong quai contains estrogen-like compounds, which should not be taken by pregnant or nursing women, children, people taking blood thinners, or people with breast cancer.

Also, dong-quai can cause photosensitivity so limit sun exposure and wear sunblock when using it.

For more about dong-quai, visit the HYPERLINK below:

http://www.herbs-wholesale.com/Dong-Quai-463.htm

Suma Brazilian Ginseng

Known as the Brazilian Ginseng, Suma is grown in Brazils Amazon Basin. The soil there is high in iron oxide and other nutrients; thus, it is assumed that the herb is high in iron because of the soil.

Suma is useful for women for anemia, fatigue and premenstrual syndrome. Look for Suma in the Natures Way Product Line at these websites:

http://www.vitacost.com/productResults.aspx?x=0& y=0&ntk=products&ss=1&Ntt=suma

http://www.luckyvitamin.com/item/itemKey/55187

Yellow Dock Root

Yellow dock root is an effective way to build up your iron stores. This herb is available dried or can be purchased as a tincture. It is effective against Anemia, liver congestion, and constipation. It also helps treat blood and skin disease. Yellow dock root can also be used as an astringent and purifier.

Yellow Dock Iron Tonic

Concocting yellow dock iron tonic is simple, and requires only a few ingredients:

- Four ounces of cut yellow dock root,
- Three pints of distilled water, and
- Three ounces of glycerin.

Prepare three pints of distilled water and boil the yellow dock root for 2 minutes. Turn down heat and let it simmer until the liquid is down to a pint. Remove from the heat and add the glycerin. Allow the tonic to cool. Bottle and keep it in a cool place, or place it in the refrigerator.

Dose: Put one tablespoon of yellow dock iron tonic into a cup of water and drink. Do this three times a day.

Yellow Dock Root Tonic 2

Preparing a yellow dock root tonic 2 is quite simple. All you need are:

Two ounces of yellow dock root,

Four tablespoons of honey, and

Two to four tablespoons of brandy.

As an alternative to honey, try blackstrap molasses instead.

Place the yellow dock root in a quart mason jar, then fill it with boiling water. Close the jar and let it sit overnight. Strain the herb material the next morning, and then discard it.

Over a low fire, steam the remaining liquid until it is reduced to about just a cup's worth. Do not boil or simmer this liquid.

Stir in the honey until it dissolves in the liquid. Bring this mixture to a boil. Pour it afterward into a container.

Add the brandy as a preservative. Close the container and store it in a cool dry place.

Dose: Take one to two tablespoons daily. You can accompany this with 20 to 50mg. of Vitamin C. For more on the yellow dock root tonic, visit this website

http://herblore.com/service/index.php?pg=info_yello w_dock_root

Ginseng

Ginseng is good for Anemia. This powerful herb provides health benefits for all parts of your body by being able to produce red blood cells, and absorb and store the iron that the body needs. Ginseng also reduces bleeding when we are cut or wounded.

This herb also improves memory and learning faculties. It lowers cholesterol, reduces the hardening of the arteries, protects the heart from oxygen deprivation, and minimizes the risk of thinning of the blood. As an antioxidant, ginseng traps cancer-causing toxins.

Ginseng is packed with minerals that fortify the body against diseases. This is a powerful herb that helps eliminate Anemia since it contains iron, manganese, copper, potassium, calcium, sulfur, magnesium, phosphorus and other trace minerals.

Bee Pollen

Bee pollen is another natural remedy for Anemia. It is packed with minerals, vitamins, and protein that will help you build your red blood cells back up.

Bee pollen contains 18 amino acids, protein, vitamins, and minerals, enzymes and co-enzymes, fatty acids and carbohydrates. It is a complete food.

Barberry Root Bark

Barberry root herb has a tonic effect on the liver as it helps remove toxic waste from the stomach and bowels. It also has mild laxative, anti-septic, antacid and diuretic actions.

This herb is perfect for Anemia since it helps rebuild body strength.

John Heinerman, in his book called Heinerman's Encyclopedia of Fruits, Vegetables, and Herbs, 1988, give two excellent herbal foods to increase your iron body stores.

"Several very good sources of iron for women, besides desiccated liver tablets, egg yolks, legumes and iron-fortified cereals, are red beetroot and Swiss chard. One to 2 level teaspoons of Pines' beet powder added to an 8-oz glass of water or juice supplies a lot of iron" He goes on to say, "As you progress in building up your blood iron content, you can simply buy tea bags of red clover or buy it in bulk in some herbal shops. Buy around an ounce or two and place a teaspoon of it in one cup of hot water. Let it sit for around 5 minutes.

From what we know about the soil of the region in which it [suma herb] grows, we may assume that this herb [Suma] is relatively high in iron… in cases of anemia, fatigue and even premenstrual syndrome to some extent, it would appear that suma is very useful for women to take... an average of 2 capsules daily helps to supplement the diet with iron."

To gain information on where to purchase these products just search on Google.

Moringa

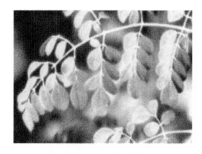

Now, here is an herb you will not normally hear about. It's called Moringa, and it's a tropical herb tree found extensively in the Philippines and in other Asian countries.

But, it is also available on the Internet quite easily.

The leaves are placed in soups, and it also comes in capsules. It has many health benefits some are:

- Kills parasites
- Combats malnutrition
- Contain more Vitamin A than Carrots
- More iron than spinach
- More Vitamin C than Oranges
- More Potassium than bananas
- High in protein

If you live where you can grow the plant or have access to this plant, then you can use the leaves in your salad or soups.

Red Clover Herb

Blood cleansing is a good idea since it helps to purify your blood. This is done by using an herbal tea called Red Clover.

Taste the tea and see if you are able to drink it without sugar. If it is too bitter, you can add a bit of honey or pure maple syrup to sweeten it. Drink a cup daily, for a week or two.

Chlorophyll

The chlorophyll, found in green leafy vegetables, is excellent for building up your blood and cleansing it. The reason it can do this is that the chlorophyll molecule is similar to that of blood. In the center of the blood molecule is iron, but by replacing the iron with magnesium, you get chlorophyll.

So by increasing the iron in your blood and taking chlorophyll supplements, you can increase the hemoglobin in your blood. This will help you reduce the effects of anemia.

Here's how to use chlorophyll. Buy liquid chlorophyll or you can buy capsules of chlorophyll. Upon waking, take one to two tablespoons of chlorophyll, more if you want, and squeeze one lemon into the chlorophyll. Then add 6 to 8 oz of water and drink it down.

The reason you should use lemon is so that it offsets the bland taste of chlorophyll. You can add chlorophyll to other juices if you like. You can just experiment to see what your taste buds like.

The foods containing high amounts of chlorophyll are:

asparagus, bell peppers, broccoli, Brussels sprouts, green cabbage, celery, collard greens, green beans, green peas, kale, leeks, green olives, parsley, romaine lettuce,

sea vegetables, spinach, Swiss chard, and turnip greens

If you are using blood thinners, then ask your doctor if you can drink chlorophyll. Chlorophyll contains vitamin k and helps to coagulate your blood when you bleed.

Red Grape Juice

Red grape juice is also another blood purifier. It helps to remove impurities from the blood. Preparing fresh grape juice is best, but as an alternative, you can buy store juices but only in glass bottles.

Colored Foods

The foods that will help you build your blood are the red vegetables and fruits. Here is a list of produce you should eat frequently.

Red apples, beets, red cabbage, cayenne pepper, red cherries, red radishes, strawberries, tomatoes, raspberries, red currants, red plums, watermelon, black cherries

Keep in mind that produce that looks like a specific organ will provide nutrients to build up that organ. That is why if a fruit or vegetable produces a red or really dark red juice, then that juice will help to build your blood.

11: Daily Supplements to Use For Anemia

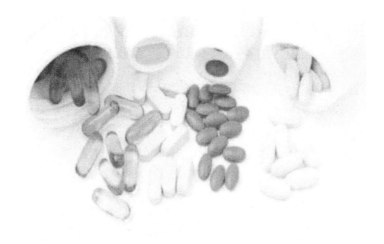

Iron Dietary Supplement

Most iron dietary supplements available today contain ferrous sulfate, a non-heme iron. Ferrous fumarate and ferrous succinate can also be found in most supplements.

Once you are diagnosed with iron deficiency, you will need to take iron supplements and iron absorption-enhancing nutrients. It is important to replenish your iron stores and build up your iron deficiency.

Iron supplements

Looking to build up your iron stores in the body? Try Enzymatic Therapy's Ultimate iron. You can order it here:

http://www.enzymatictherapy.com/Products/Energy/ Daily-Energy/05229-Ultimate-Iron.aspx

The Enzymatic Iron Supplements contains succinate iron, Vitamins B12 and C, folic acid, and fat-soluble chlorophyll. These are most of the factors that you need to build up your iron stores as well as increase the number red blood cells your body needs.

Native Remedies offers AnemiCare, a Homeopathic remedy that increases iron absorption. Here's the link to the AnemiCare page on the Native Remedies website:

http://www.nativeremedies.com/products/anemicare normal-iron-hemoglobin- levels.html?kbid=1028&sub=AffToolsSpecialBox#ingr edients

AnemiCare contains Ferrum Phos, Calcium Phos, and Ferrum metallicum, a metal essential in the formation of hemoglobin in red blood cells.

Biological Transmutation

In his book, How to Get Well, Paavo Airola, PH.D., discusses biological transmutation:

"According to Lois Kervran, the most effective way to get iron into the system (in iron-deficiency anemia) is not by taking an iron supplement, but a manganese supplement, or manganese-rich foods, such as whole grains, especially buckwheat, wheat, brown or red rice, beans, etc. By biological transmutation, manganese changes in the body into iron the form of iron that is easily assimilated and used by the body."

Vitamin Supplements

Vitamin supplements help prevent iron deficiency. Here is a list of vitamins and nutrients that will help increase your iron stores, and prevent iron deficiency:

- High potency B10Vitamins
- PABA (up to 5mg.)
- Vitamin E (up to 100IU)
- Crude blackstrap molasses (at least 2 tbsp.)
- Bone meal (3 tablets)
- Sesame seeds (Add them to your salads or smoothies)
- Vitamin C (at least 50mg.)
- Kelp
- Manganese
- Betaine hydrochloride

In addition to High potency B10Vitamins, supply yourself with the following:

- Folic acid (0. 5 to 1 mg.)
- Vitamin B12 (25 to 5mcg.)
- Vitamin B6 (5to 10mg.)
- Pantothenic Acid (up to 10mg.)

Moreover, 50 mg of Vitamin C promotes the absorption of iron in the body, but take more vitamin C, like 1000 mg. On the other hand, betaine hydrochloride adds HCl acid to your stomach, which in turn helps in the assimilation of Iron and Vitamin B12.

There are many vitamins and minerals that are involved in making, building, and maintaining red blood cells. The main nutrients that you cannot be short on are iron, Vitamin B12, and folic acid. Here is a list of additional supplements that you need to take:

- Vitamin C,

- Vitamin E,

- Zinc,

- Vitamin K and Fish Oil,

- copper

If you chose a different iron supplement, you may experience side effects, such as nausea, digestive discomfort, and constipation. If this happens, use them with your meals or get your prescription lowered.

Iron supplements should be recommended by your doctor, and the best type to use is iron succinate. This type of iron supplement has very few reports of side effects.

Alert: Excessive iron supplementation can cause massive free-radical reactions, which set into motion diseases like cancer, heart disease, and neurological degeneration. So always take iron supplements under a doctor's care.

Other types of iron used in the treatment of mild to moderate iron Deficiency Anemia are Iron(II) sulfate ferrous sulfate or ferrous gluconate.

http://en.wikipedia.org/wiki/Iron%28II%29_sulfate

o

Vitamin C

Vitamin C plays an important part in how much iron you absorb. The more Vitamin C you have in your digestive system and body, the more iron you will absorb.

You can get plenty of vitamin C from fruits and vegetables. Thus, it is important to eat fruits and vegetables.

To get the Vitamin C you need for Anemia, take 500 to 1000 mg daily. Break up this amount in three or four quantities during the day.

Vitamin C can cause gas or diarrhea, and if it does, back off slightly on the amount you are taking. Return to the same dose the next day. Do this until you are able to take up to 500 mg of Vitamin C per day.

In their book, The Healing Foods, 1989, Patricia Hausman and Judith Benn Hurley report,

"In the plant world, iron's best friend is Vitamin C. In their classic paper on iron absorption, Elaine Monsen, Ph. D., and co-workers reported that the iron in a meal is well absorbed as long as 75 milligrams of Vitamin C are also present. As an alternative, said Dr. Monsen, even a modest size serving, 3 oz., of meat, poultry, or fish, will also make the iron in a meat highly absorbable, [with Vitamin C]."

Here is a list of vegetables and fruits that can give you 75 mg. of Vitamin C, so eat them to make the iron you eat more absorbable.

Foods with 75 mg of Vitamin C

- 1 cup broccoli
- 1 cup Brussels sprouts
- ½ cantaloupe
- 1 cup cauliflower
- 1cup collard greens
- A cup cranberry juice cocktail
- 1 cup grapefruit juice (fresh or from concentrate)
- 1 cup kale
- 1 cup orange juice (fresh or from concentrate)
- 1 cup of papaya chunks
- 1 cup pineapple juice
- 1 cup fresh strawberries
- ½ package frozen strawberries (10-ounce package)

Vitamin C is also an antioxidant that will help neutralize free radicals in the body. Free radicals cause illnesses that are likely to develop, from heart disease to cancer.

Taking Vitamin C also helps increase bone density and health. Since red blood cells are produced by bone marrow, keeping your bones healthy will keep the production of red blood cells active.

Another reason to eat citrus fruits and sauerkraut, aside from its Vitamin C content, is their acid content. Citric acid helps the absorption of iron in your body.

Vitamin E

Vitamin E is a good protection against heart disease and cancer. Take up to 40 IU daily.

A deficiency in vitamin E is rare. However, there is a correlation between Anemia and Vitamin E deficiency. Those who are diagnosed as anemic are also found to be

deficient in Vitamin E.

Folic Acid

Folic acid is needed for blood cell replication, growth, and regeneration. Fruits, vegetables, and grains are high in folic acid. If you do not eat plenty of these daily, you may not be getting the 40 mcg. of folic acid recommended by the FDA.

Severe folic deficiency is rare, but mild to borderline conditions may exist in many individuals. The elderly are at risk for folic deficiency since they:

- eat more cooked food, which loses the folic acid
- use more drugs anticonvulsant, anticancer, cortisone, sleeping pills, or sulfa drugs - that interfere with folate nutrition

- lack the ability to absorb folate from food as they age
- can deplete their folic acid quickly

Generally, you cannot get the amount of folic acid you need by increasing your intake of fruits and vegetables. You will need to take a folic acid supplement.

Folic acid works with 2 different enzymes to make your DNA -the material that contains your genetic code.

Folic acid also plays an important role in the development of babies. Folic acid deficiency can produce life-threatening defects in the brain and spine. This defect usually occurs during the first two weeks of pregnancy.

Another benefit of folic acid is that it helps prevent arteriosclerosis, hardening of the arteries, by changing the harmful amino acid homocysteine into a formless damaging to the arteries.

Using birth control pills can reduce folic acid in the body, as well as Vitamin B12. Doctors recommend a minimum of 40 mcg. of folic acid daily.

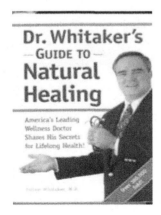

In Dr. Whitaker's Guide to Natural Healing, 1995, he talks about what he recommends to his anemic patients, "When I need to prescribe an iron supplement, I usually use **Enzymatic Therapy's Ultimate Iron.**

Each capsule contains 30 mg of ferrous succinate and 250 mg of liquid live fractions. Ultimate iron provides highly absorbable iron and is relatively free from side effects like nausea, constipation, or diarrhea, common to other iron supplements. Ultimate Iron includes the liver fractions rich in 'heme' iron...

While heme iron is absorbed intact, non-heme is dependent upon ionization and complex transport mechanisms. A breakdown of these mechanisms can harm your body's ability to uptake non-heme iron.

In addition, non-hem iron is extremely susceptible to blocking agents, such as fiber, phosphates, calcium, tannates, and preservatives. Heme iron is not affected by these factors."

12: Minerals and Vitamin B12 for Low Iron Blood

Vitamin B12 Deficiency Triggers Anemia

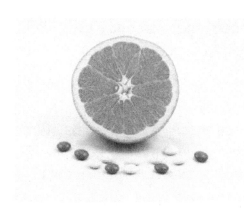

When the level of Vitamin B12 is reduced to that below what is needed in the body, a vitamin deficiency results. This is largely due to the lack of iron nutritional diet.

Consequently, a Vitamin B12 Deficiency also triggers Iron Deficiency Anemia.

Iron Deficiency Anemia is due to the insufficient intake, or absorption of iron. It includes the failure to replace losses from menstruation or from diseases. Since iron is an essential element in hemoglobin, its low levels will result in a weakened incorporation of hemoglobin in red blood cells.

In pre-menopausal women, blood is lost during their menstrual periods. Accordingly, the resulting iron deficiency, especially in teenage girls, causes poor performance in school.

On a worldwide scale, iron deficiency is the most prevalent deficiency state.

Iron Deficiency Anemia is also due to the bleedings lesions of the gastrointestinal tract. Through fecal occult blood testing or upper and lower endoscopies, these bleeding lesions are detected and identified.

In men and post-menopausal women, there are higher chances that the bleeding lesions in their gastrointestinal tract could be caused by colon polyp or colorectal cancer.

Parasitic infestation is also regarded as one of the most common causes of iron deficiency around the world. Hookworms, whipworms, amebiasis, and schistosomiasis are among the guilty parasites.

There is also a link between pregnancy and iron deficiency. Pregnant women lose about two milligrams of iron every day, totaling to around during their pregnancy. To replenish the lost iron, they need to take iron supplements.

Vitamin B12, on the other hand, is used to make red blood cells in the bone marrow. B12 injections may be necessary, in case B12 capsules have no significant effect.

Trace minerals also help reduce the effect of Anemia on normal blood cell functions. These are:

- Copper (at 2mg.),
- Zinc (at 3mg.), and
- Selenium (at 20mg.)

Fish oil and Vitamin K also help reduce inflammatory molecules that attack the red blood cells.

Copper

Gary Nulls book called, Power Aging, 2003 discusses copper,

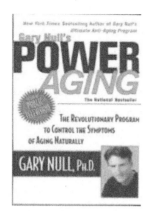

"Trace amounts of copper are present in all human tissues, but copper is most concentrated in your liver, kidneys, brain, bones, and muscles, and it is essential in blood. Copper increases iron assimilation. Copper and iron form hemoglobin and red blood cells.

In fact, anemia can be a symptom of a copper deficiency."

Some of the symptoms of a copper deficiency are:

- allergies,
- Parasites,
- Parkinson's disease,
- Reduced glucose tolerance,
- Aneurysms,
- Arthritis,
- Dry brittle hair
- Hernias
- High blood cholesterol,
- Thyroid issues
- Hair loss
- Liver cirrhosis,
- Heart disease, varicose veins,
- Skin eruptions

Zinc

Zinc is useful for cell production. It helps create new cells needed for healing, growth, or during pregnancy.

When one is wounded or cut, zinc helps replicate cells quickly by creating collagen to heal the wound fast.

During their menstrual period, women can be irritable and give off the stay-away-from-me reaction. Zinc helps them normalize their mood.

Second, only to calcium, Zinc is the most deficient mineral in a woman's diet. Thus, women need to supplement it with at least 15 mg. of zinc every day.

The nutritional body requirements

What is important to understand is that deficiencies in any one vitamin or mineral do not create an iron deficiency. It is the cascade of chemical changes that occur when that one vitamin or mineral is lacking.

This cascade idea is well put by Dr. Michael Colgan in his book called Hormonal Health, 1996, when he said,

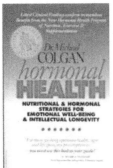

"Vitamin E deficiency also depletes your body of zinc, despite ample zinc in your diet. When E is low, zinc pinch-hits for some of its functions, thereby rising your zinc requirement. Without sufficient zinc to control it, body levels of copper then increase to cause all sorts of toxic mischief.

Another example is vitamin B6, which a recent government study showed was deficient in 80% of a representative sample of 38,000 Americans. Vitamin B6 deficiency impairs vitamin B2 metabolism which, in turn, impairs folic acid metabolism.

Folic acid dysfunction then impairs Vitamin C metabolism, which then reduces body absorption of iron, which allows excess copper absorption, which impairs zinc metabolism, and so on and on and on."

This is one of the reasons nutritionist recommend taking a multivitamin and mineral supplement.

13: A 7 Day Meal Program for Iron Deficiency Blood

Lunch and Dinner Meal Suggestions

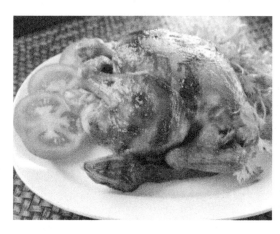

Here are some meals that will give you more iron. By adding Vitamin C-rich foods, you will absorb and digest iron at an increased rate.

If you don't have the fruits, for vitamin C, then take a good vitamin C, general vitamin, and mineral supplement.

Breakfast meal ideas have already been given in the previous chapter. Here are some lunch and dinner ideas. Use them as a base and add those other iron foods listed in this e-book to these recipes.

Day 1:

Lunch

3 ounces chicken breast (without skin)

2 slices Italian bread

1 cup honeydew melon

1 cup skim milk

Green salad with vegetable high in iron

Snack

1 red apple

1-ounce cheddar cheese

Dinner

1 cup oyster

¾ cup cooked eggplant

1 ½ cups raw celery

1 cup raw green pepper

1 fresh tomato

1 cup fresh pineapple chunks with ½ cup vanilla
low-fat yogurt

Day 2:

Lunch

¾ cup fresh spinach

6 cucumber slices (with peel)

1 fresh tomato

3 ounces steamed scallops

¼ cup seedless raisins

¼ cup pumpkin seeds

1 cup skim milk

Snack

1 apple

1-ounce cheddar cheese

Dinner

4 ounces chicken breast (without skin)

1 simmered chicken liver

½ cup peas

½ cup brown rice

1 cup pineapple juice

Day 3:

Lunch

2 ounces water-packed tuna

½ tablespoon reduced-calorie mayonnaise

½ cup canned peas

½ cup butterhead lettuce

1 fresh tomato

1 tablespoon low-calorie salad dressing

1 cup skim milk

Snack

½ cup fresh orange sections

Dinner

2 ½ ounces lean sirloin steak (trimmed of fat)

1/3 cup unsweetened applesauce

1 cup lima beans

½ tablespoon margarine

1 cup skim milk

1-ounce black walnuts

Day 4:

Lunch

3 ounces ground round patty with 1 slice low-fat   cheese

1 ½ cups tossed salad

2 tablespoons low-calorie salad dressing

2 pieces of Italian bread

1 cup tomato juice

Snack

1 cup fresh strawberries with ½ cup vanilla low-fat yogurt

Dinner

4 ounces Cornish hen (without skin)

1 whole wheat roll

¾ cup Brussels sprouts

1 tablespoon margarine

1 cup skim milk

1 cup cantaloupe

Day 5:

Lunch

1 cup fresh spinach (limit the frequency of eating this veggie)

¼ cup dry bread crumbs

9 cucumber slices (with peel)

1 apple

1 cup raw broccoli

½ cup raw cauliflower

2 tablespoons low-calorie salad dressing

1 cup low-fat yogurt

Snack½ cup dates, raisins, or prunes

Dinner

2 simmered chicken livers

¼ cup onions

½ cup brown rice

½ cup Great Northern beans

1 cup skim milk

½ tablespoon margarine

1 piece watermelon

Day 6:

Lunch

1 cup fresh spinach

½ cup green beans

½ cup navy beans

2 pieces tofu (soybean curd)

6 cucumber slices (with peel)

1/3 raw celery

¼ cup shredded cheese

2 tablespoons low-calorie salad dressing

Snack

¼ cup raisin-nut mix

Dinner

3 ounces veal cutlet

½ cup mashed potatoes

1 cup peas

1 tablespoon margarine

¾ orange juice

1 cup fresh raspberries with ½ cup frozen low-fat yogurt

Day 7:

Lunch

2 tomatoes stuffed with 1 cup canned clams, ½ cup low-fat

cottage cheese, 1 tablespoon

reduced-calorie mayonnaise

¾ cup orange juice

Snack

½ cup dried apricots

Dinner

3 ounces calves' liver

½ lima beans

1 small boiled potato

1 tablespoon margarine

1 cup skim milk

1 cup fresh strawberries

Fruits should not be eaten with your meals wait at least 1/2 hour or more after your meal to eat fruit.

Use some of the other foods listed in this e-book to make your meals, these are just suggested meals. By concentrating on foods that are high in iron, you will start to build up your body iron stores.

14: Three Natural Body Cycles to Increase your Blood Iron

Natural Body Cycles

Here is a way of eating to maintain your health and to prevent

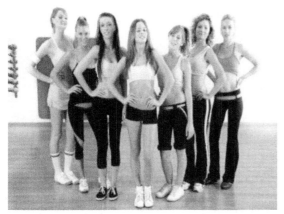

disease. It is a method to help you work with the cycles in your body. Your body does

things in cycles and if you know what these cycles are, you can enhance your health by helping your body do what it knows to do and when it knows to do it.

This eating method can help your body absorb and process the food you eat in a more efficient way. In this way, you will get more benefit from the food you eat. The iron food you eat will be used as intended and not wasted by your body's inefficiency, as a result of not having a healthy body.

Your body has three cycles. It has an internal body regeneration and toxic removal time or cycle. Then it has a time where it wants to eliminate the accumulated toxic matter from your body. And, finally, it has a time that it needs to intake food for cycle regeneration and daily functioning.

This first thing to know is that your last meal must be taken at least three hours before your bedtime. The heavier the meal the more time you should give your body to process this food before bedtime.

Your body uses sleep time to regenerate itself and process unfinished digested food. It goes through various organs to cleanse them and detoxify them. If you provide your body with the proper food for these processes, it will do it a job better.

First Body Cycle 6 am to noon

By the early morning, when you are ready to get up, the toxins and chemicals your body has gathered are in the form of urine or fecal matter. Your body now needs your help to remove this collected matter out of your body.

The longer this matter stays in your body the more toxic it is and the more stress your body goes through trying to keep those toxins inside your body. Even if you do not feel the need for a bowel movement, the stress is still there.

For some of you, your first instinct is to urinate and have a bowel movement. For those of you that are not like that, then this is the way to help your body.

Once you are up, do not have a typical breakfast. A breakfast of solid food disrupts the elimination cycle your body has in mind. You need to drink only water, fruit or vegetable juices, or eat fruit.

Doing this doesn't disrupt your first natural cycle. Your body wants to eliminate in the morning, but any heavy food stops this process because your body now has to concentrate on digesting the food in your stomach, instead of setting up to have a bowel movement.

Having liquid for breakfast will help you promote a bowel movement. First liquids or fruits only take an hour or so to be digested whereas solid food can take up to 3 to 4 hours and by that time lunch has come around.

Second, by choosing the right juices, you give your body a boost by stimulating the peristaltic action of your large intestine. Here are some drinks to make or buy.

Make a lemon drink by squeezing two lemons into the blender with 6 or so oz. of water. Then add a pinch of cayenne powder and honey to your taste. Drink this every morning to stimulate your liver and kidney to detoxify more.

Another morning drink is buying liquid chlorophyll and putting one tablespoon into 6 oz of water. Add the juice of one lemon and drink up. Chlorophyll is high in iron and is also a colon, body and blood detoxifier.

Buy pure tomato juice and add the juice of one lemon. Any red vegetable or fruit will build your red blood cells.

Drink a glass of prune juice to get your bowels moving and to give yourself some extra iron.

Drinking a glass of cherry, grapefruit, orange, or any other juice you find can activate a bowel movement.

Fruits are also great in the morning. Those fruits with more juice are most helpful since they are digested quicker than fruits that are more solid. Use watermelon, cantaloupes, peaches, cherries, mango, or banana.

Experiment with different juices and fruits to see which ones your body needs. Your body knows what nutrients it needs; that is why you like some fruits over others and at different times.

Second Body Cycle Noon to 6 pm

Here is the time when you can have a great meal. You have eliminated all the waste your body has collected during the night and now its time to replenish your body.

First of all every heavy meal you eat you should always have some raw vegetables or slightly cooked ones to complement your main course.

If you eat meat or carbohydrate such as rice, potatoes, noodles, these foods do not have fiber. You need fiber to help process and digest these foods so that during the night cleansing cycle these digested foods will be ready to come out the next day.

Do not have any liquid or ice drinks with your meals. You can drink some water when food accumulates in your throat. Drinking liquids with your meal dilute your stomach acids and this will cause incomplete digestion of your food. This will also cause you not to get the most iron you need from your foods.

Third Body Cycle6 pm to 6 am

The last body cycle is from your last meal to bedtime. Try to keep your dinner meals lighter than your lunch meal. The reason is that you don't want your body to be digesting your food during the night when it should be cleansing and detoxifying your body.

For a heavy meal, it will take four hours or so to get digested in the stomach and then sent on to the lower intestines. So, by taking your meals around 6 to 7 pm and heading to bed around 1 to 10:3, you give your body time to digest your food.

By midnight and after, your body is busy cleaning you out and preparing for elimination in the morning cycle. Don't block this process with a heavy morning breakfast.

15: Some Final Comments On Anemia

There are many foods that have iron, but each one of them is

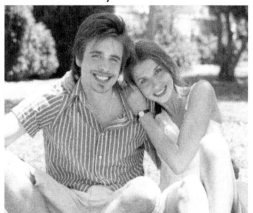

not enough to supply you with the iron you need if you have an iron deficiency.

That is why you need to have an "Iron plan" that will give you the iron your body needs and to replenish your body's

iron supplies.

Your plan should consist of getting the iron from the various food sources listed in this e-book. In addition, you should be taking those vitamins that are required to improve your absorption of iron.

You should follow those ideas and techniques that give you better absorption of iron.

And you should take the minerals that give your body a chance to utilize the iron you eat. Keep in mind the use of the transmutation manganese supplement. Re-read this about this mineral if you forgot what it does.

Study the different herbs that help you gain body iron and buy those herbs in crushed leaves, powder, or roots. Mix these herbs in equal parts and make an herb tea. Place one teaspoon or tablespoon of these mixed herbs into a glass of hot water and let it sit from 5 to 10 minutes. Add a little honey, if necessary, and drink it down. The longer you let them sit before you drink it, the strong it will be, and that's ok if you can bear the strong taste.

You can use a glass of tea or two every day until you restore your iron levels.

You have plenty of information in this book to get yourself back to good health. Don't be afraid to experiment with the information you have here. It's your body, and you need to take control of what your health iron plan will be.

And last, make sure you use the body cycles to restore your body's health so that you can get back to normal, and improve your immune system.

16: The Author and Resources

Rudy Silva is a natural nutritional consultant educated in the United States in Nutrition and Physics.   He is a graduate of San Jose State University in California. He is the author of 40 other books on natural remedies.   He has authored a newsletter in natural remedies for over 10 years.

Resource page

To see all of the books written by this author, go to the Google and type in the keyword, Rudy Silva.

If you need support or want to promote any of his e-books, please contact him at rss41@yahoo.com.

Give A Review

And, don't forget to give a review of this book. It's not hard to give a review. It can be only a sentence or two. You don't have to leave a long review. A short review helps other people decide if they want to buy a book. So give a short review and give your thoughts to help other people and to help the author improve his book.

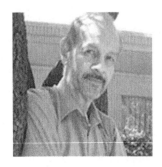

To you, for creating better health and more happiness,

Rudy S Silva

Printed in Great Britain
by Amazon

17845008R00078